EASY TO LEARN SEXUAL MASSAGE

A Brief Guide to Yoni and Lingam Massage

by Deborah Glass

Copyright 2014

*Dedicated to
my Husband, Ron*

THE YONI MASSAGE

BACKGROUND INFORMATION

Yoni (pronounced YO-KNEE) is a Sanskrit word for the vagina that could be loosely translated as the "Sacred Temple." It's meaning in Sanskrit is in contrast to the alternate perspective of the Westerner's view of the female genitalia, many names of which may or may not be complimentary depending on the intent of their usage. In Tantra, the Yoni is seen from a perspective of pure love, trust and respect, which is helpful for men, as well as women, to learn.

The purpose of the Yoni Massage is to create a space for the woman (the receiver) to relax, and enter a state of high stimulation and experience deep pleasure from the Yoni. Her partner (the provider) experiences the pleasure of being of service and observing a special moment for one experiencing. The Yoni Massage can also be used as a type of safe-r sex (when rubber gloves are used) and is a fantastic activity to build intimacy and trust. Many sex and massage therapists use it to assist breaking through trauma and sexual blockages.

Although it is often a welcome side effect, the overall purpose of Yoni massage is not orgasm. The purpose is simply to massage and enjoy the Yoni, or vagina. This way both the woman receiving and person providing can be at ease, and not have to worry about anything except achieving exceptional enjoyment. If an orgasm does occur (and usually it will) it is most likely to be more drawn out, expanded, satisfying and intense than a climax not using Yoni massage. Either way, you must allow orgasm to happen or not happen.

It is also helpful for the provider to expect nothing in return. As the provider you must learn to allow the receiver to freedom to enjoy the massage, and to relax deeply into her self when it is finished. Granted, other forms of sexuality or activity may follow, but always this should be the receiver's decision. If this acknowledged before hand it will build greater trust, intimacy and compassion, and has the potential to expand your sexual awareness.

PREPARATION:

First, prepare a warm bath as it is always beneficial for clearing away the energy of the day and will relax both people involved. A peaceful space should be chosen with soft music, warm candles, and comfortable pillows, and whatever else would bring those involved a relaxed and safe feeling. You should allow enough time, never rushing or hurrying through the entire practice.

Please note to always use the bathroom before this kind of massage. For the best experience the bowels and bladder should be emptied, and this will circumvent the unnecessary occurrence of interrupting a massage to use the restroom.

Warm up to your partner by creating trust and intimacy by hugging, holding each other, gazing into each other's eyes for an extended time, or anything else that brings you a sense of safety and assurance.

PROCEDURE:

Have the woman receiving the massage lie down on her back, preferably with a pillow underneath the head so she can have a comfortable view of her genitals and also at her partner. Also, place a towel-covered pillow underneath her hips, with her legs spread apart with the knees slightly bent and genitals openly exposed and ready for massage.

The provider should sit between the receiver's legs, cross-legged. The provider may choose to be seated on a pillow as well. This will allow complete access to the woman's Yoni and also the rest of the body.

Before a single touch occurs, both participants should start with relaxed and deep breathing. By breathing slowly and deeply with the intention of full relaxation, both parties will help to relax each other deepening the emotional connection as well as the physical. The provider should calmly remind the receiver if she begins to take shallower breaths. Deep, relaxed breathing is quite important to this process.

Slowly and gently begin to massage the feet, the calves, the legs and thighs, buttocks, back, breasts, and more in order to have the receiver continue to relax and for the provider to prepare for the nurturing of the Yoni. You may also pour a small amount of quality lubricant or oil to spread on the Yoni's mound. Use enough to that it seeps down from the outside lips and lubricates the entire outside of the Yoni. (There are many online stores that carry high-quality vaginal lubrication)

Now you begin touching the Yoni by starting with a gentle massage of the mound and outer lips. Take your time and avoid rushing the process. Slowly and lovingly give the massage and give pleasure with every long stroke. Squeeze the outer lip gently using the thumb and index finger, sliding back and forth through the entirety of both lips. Repeat the same process on the inner lips, carefully stroking while taking as long as needed to build pleasure. You can also massage the area outside and around the outer lips as this stimulates additional wetness from the receiver.

The receiver can just relax and continue deep breathing, or may add to the massage by gently massaging her own breasts. It can also be beneficial for the provider to lubricate the nipples of the receiver as well.

It is good for both parties involved to maintain rapport by gazing into each others eyes, preferably as much as possible although as the massage continues this can lessen considerably, especially as the woman seems to approach orgasm. Still, the receiver may let the provider know if the depth, pressure, or speed of the massage should be decreased or increased. Keep the talking at a minimum and focus the intent on having pleasing sensations.

When there is too much speaking this tends to diminish the effect of the massage.

Using soft motions at first, stroke the clitoris gently in a clockwise, then counter-clockwise motion. Begin to gently squeeze the clit with the index finger and thumb. Remember, this is a massage and not just quick stroking for the receiver to "get off." Take your time, and enjoy sensing the receiver becoming very aroused. Encourage her to breathe, relax and enjoy the stimulation.

After she is considerably aroused, you may insert the middle finger of the right hand inside the Yoni. Do this very slowly at first, and with great care. Always use the right hand instead of the left, because in Tantra the right hand gives energy, as opposed to the left, which receives it. Slowly explore and massage the inner Yoni with the middle finger. Always remember to be gentle, take your time, and move in all directions (up, down, sideways) and do it with great care.

As you massage, make subtle changes in the speed, depth, and pressure of the massage. The idea is to nurture and relax the Yoni as much as possible.

Now with your palm up, and middle finger within the Yoni, glide the middle finger in a "come hither" motion, crooking back the palm of the hand. Your finger will make contact with spongy tissue right under the pubic bone directly behind the clitoris. This is what is known as the "G-Spot," and in Tantra it is known as the "Sacred Spot." The receiver will most likely find this very pleasurable, although they also may feel some pain or a sensation as if they have to urinate. Like before, vary the speed, pressure and pattern of movement. You move in circles, back and forth, or side to side with the middle finger. At this point a second finger may also be inserted, the ring finger between the middle and pink. Respectfully ask your partner if she would like this before bringing the second finger inside of her. Most of the time women will not object and very much enjoy the additional stimulation of a second finger. Be gentle, take your time and keep the mood relaxed. Additionally, you may rub with the thumb of the right hand to give stimulation to the clitoris as well.

Another option you may try if the receiver is comfortably with it is inserting the right hand pink finger into the hole of anus. Always ask first and never insert the pinky finger into the Yoni after it has visited the anus. Lubrication should always be used and a gentle approach is greatly emphasized here.

There is a saying in Tantra, that when the thumb is upon the clitoris, the middle and ring finger inside the Yoni, and the pinky within the anus, that One is "holding one of the great secrets of the Universe in your hand."

Concerning the left hand, you may use it to do several different things, including the massaging of the breasts, touching of the abdomen or additional stimulation of the clitoris. When massaging the clitoris a good technique to use is your thumb in an up and down motion, while the base of the hand rests on and massages the mound. The double stimulation of using both hands provides must pleasure for the on receiving. Stimulation of the provider's genitals is not recommended as it removes the focus from the receiver—the basis for this massage is the heightened pleasure and physical stimulation of the receiver only. Keeping this intent will increase the pleasure a thousand fold.

Continue the massage, varying the speeds and patterns of movement as well as the pressure. Try to continue gazing into the other's eyes. The woman may end up having very powerful emotions, even crying. If this occurs continue breathing and stay on her with a gentle touch. Some women have been abused sexually in the past and are in need of healing. Being a loving, patient, and giving partner can be a much-needed source of comfort for her.

If the receiver begins to orgasm, continue breathing, and continue to massage her if she is clear this is what she wants. The first orgasm also might not be her last, because in Tantric sexual massage more orgasms can occur. This practice is called "riding a wave" and many women can become multi-orgasmic with Yoni Massage and a loving partner.

Continue the massage until she gives you the sign to stop. Now gently, slowly, and with love and respect, remove the hands from her Yoni. Give her space to lie and enjoy the glow of a completely Yoni massage. As you practice the Yoni massage more and you will eventually become Master of your own sex life, and you will be greatly enriched by what you will learn about women and their sexuality.

Similarly, there is a massage that is for men that is called "Lingam Massage." In the Sanskrit language Lingam is the word for penis that translates to "the Wand of Light."

THE LINGAM MASSAGE

BACKGROUND INFORMATION

In Sanskrit the word for penis is Lingam (pronounced LING-AM) and can be roughly translated as the "Wand of Light." It's meaning is different in intention from the typical Western view of the penis. In Tantric practice and Sacred Sexuality, the Lingam is respected and honored, as the "Wand of Light" is the channel for pleasure and creative energies.

The idea of Lingam Massage is to create space for the receiver to relax and enjoy drawn out pleasure from the Lingam. His partner or "provider" is allowed to experience the pleasure of giving, while witnessing the surrender of the man to his gentle, nurturing side. It can also be a form of safe-r sex (when rubber gloves are used) and is a fantastic process to build intimacy and trust with a partner. Many times it can be used for sexual healing from negative conditioning or sexual trauma.

Like Yoni massage, we are not massaging the Lingam for the goal of orgasm. Still, it can be a pleasurable side effect of the massage. The focus is the massage of the Lingam, testicles, perineum and what is known as the "Sacred Spot" which is male equivalent of the woman's G-spot. This is a way for the man to surrender to a type of pleasure he might not be used to. Both the provider and receiver will need to be very relaxed to enjoy the extended pleasure of this type of massage.

Considering that most Western-male conditioning has the man in a goal-oriented and giving sexual function, the purpose of Lingam is for the man to receive and relax. This allows the receiver to experience his softer receptive side and experience a new kind of pleasure that differs from the traditional perspective.

PREPARATION:

Have a warm and relaxing shower or bath. Try to take your time, breathe deeply and get relaxed. Some deep breathing will help take both of you out of the over-thinking mind and get you both in touch with your feelings. Relax the belly and release tension that might be held there.

Like the Yoni massage, use the restroom before beginning the massage. For best results make sure the bladder and bowels are empty.

Let go of your thoughts and connect with your partner through hugging, holding, eye gazing (looking into each other's eyes for an extended time), bringing both of you to a place of relaxation and trust.

Warm up to your partner by creating trust and intimacy by hugging, holding each other, staring into each other's eyes for an extended time, or anything else that brings you both a sense of safety and assurance.

PROCEDURE:

Have the man receiving the massage lie down on his back, preferably with a pillow underneath the head so she can have a comfortable view of his genitals and also of his partner. Also, place a towel-covered pillow underneath the hips, with legs spread apart with the knees slightly bent and genitals openly exposed and ready for massage.

The giver will sit cross-legged between the legs of the receiver. Before touching the body, start the massage with full, relaxed breathing. Massage the legs, thighs, chest, abdomen, nipples and more to give the receiver more time to relax. Keep reminding the receiver to breathe deeply and to fully relax, which is key to creating the best possible Lingam massage.

Begin by pouring a small amount of quality lubricant on the shaft of the Lingam, as well as the testicles. Start to gently massage and tug the testicles, and use care to cause no pain in this very sensitive area. Next, gently massage the scrotum, allowing it to relax. Massage the area directly above the Lingam in the area of the pubic bone. Massage the area between the testicles and anus. Always go slow, take your time and remember that you are providing a massage to an often neglected part of the body.

Handle the shaft, massaging the Lingam up and down. Change the speed and pressure while gently squeezing at the base with the right hand. Pull the Lingam up, slide off, then alternate with the other hand. Again, take your time while doing this, alternating between right, left, right, left. Next, change directions and squeeze at the head of the Lingam, sliding DOWN and off. Alternate this process with right and left hands.

Massage and gently pump the head of the Lingam as if you were using a fruit juicer. Continue the massage all around the top of the head and down the shaft. In Tantric sexuality is is known that there are thousands of nerve endings that correspond to other parts of the body, all upon the Lingam. In fact it is believed that receiving a Lingam massage can heal many ailments.

Please note that the Lingam become soft as you are performing the technique. Do not worry if it does not harden again right away. Most likely it will get hard, then become soft, harden again, back and forth, which in Tantra is a highly desirable experience, the equivalent of "riding a wave." Keep in mind that being hard and being soft are both ends of the same pleasure spectrum.

If it seems as if the receiver is about to ejaculate, slow down and back off pressure, and allow the Lingam to slightly soften before resuming the massage. Repeat this a few times, getting close to ejaculation, and then easing off. Keep in mind the purpose is not orgasm by itself. A man can learn the art of mastering ejaculation and stay in control by being close to ejaculation and then easing off from the stimulation. Stick with breathing deeply and this will lessen the urge to ejaculate. Eventually mastering ejaculation will permit you to make love as long as you would like and become multi-orgasmic without losing one drop of semen. Soon you will find that ejaculation and orgasms are two different things you can learn to separate. This will expand your sex life as a result.

Next, you can find, and then massage, the Sacred Spot. There are two main ways to do this. The first way is by locating the spot halfway between the anus and testicles. You will find a small indentation roughly the size of a pea, possibly maybe larger. Be very gentle and begin to push inward. The man will feel a deep pressure inside of him, and it may be very painful when you first begin. As the Sacred Spot is worked with and softened, the man will be able to extend his orgasms and master his own ejaculatory control.

Massaging the Lingam with your right hand and massaging his Sacred Spot with your left hand will bring him incredible pleasure. Also, try to push in on the spot when he is close to ejaculation.

Another way to reach the Sacred Spot is through his anus, although many men, especially men who are heterosexual, can be uncomfortable with this at first. This can be because of sexual conditioning of a negative nature. Be sure to take care of and remove any hangnails you might have before hand as they can be very excruciating for the man. Use good judgment here, be careful and use plenty of lubrication. The idea is to move slowly and be gentle. Insure that he is breathing when you slip a finger from the left hand into his anus, only about an inch or less. Next arch the finger back in a "come hither" gesture. With this movement, you will feel the prostate gland. Be sure to vary the pressure and change speed of massage as needed. He will mostly likely require stimulation of his Lingam when you massage the Sacred Spot. As he approaches orgasm ease off from the Lingam and increase pressure on the Sacred Spot.

Occasionally a man may feel powerful emotions during your access to his Sacred Spot. The man may cry, or recall a traumatizing event from the past. You, as the provider, should continue to nurture and stay in a place of trust and intimacy. Allow him to feel the emotions his is having, going out of your way to be loving. Avoid trying to console him, just allow him to feel whatever he needs to feel. You may encourage him to cry, scream, moan or even sob if it feels right for the situation. Your job is to be the healer and friend in that moment.

ENDING THE MASSAGE:

If the man decides to let go completely and ejaculate, encourage deep breathing during his orgasm. This will surely blow his mind, and works especially well if he has come close and then held himself from ejaculating at least SIX times. When a man holds back six times it charges up his "sexual batteries" with an awesome energy. Then it is up to him as to where he would like to send his energy -- out with their semen (most common for men) or inward for other purposes (men who master their ejaculations can channel the energy into other areas of themselves).

When the man feels complete and feeling finished with your massage carefully remove your hands and let him lie quietly until he feels done with his session. You can always get close together or you can even leave the room to allow him to be in a meditative state. Allow him whatever he needs to fully experience his true innocence and magnificence of manhood.

Be sure to share the techniques in this book with your friends and loved ones!